The Ultimate Keto Diet Book For Beginners

Quick and Delicious Recipes For a Whole Lifestyle incl. Breakfast, Main and Side Dishes

Matthew Hollandar

ISBN - [9798775849658]

TABLE OF CONTENTS

Are you looking for the right diet for YOU? Are you looking to change up your lifestyle drastically, freshen things up, or build muscle gains? Either way, this book will show you why the ketogenic option is right for you. Even if you are simply considering the diet, or just want to know more about it, then look no further than this book, where we lay out the basics; the benefits, the risks, and a host of easy to make meals.

What is ketosis? In a nutshell, it is a metabolic state where your body fuels itself with fat instead of carbs. Does that sound too simple to make a significant difference? Well, when the body enters into this process a whole host of benefits open up. Would you have guessed that the mere process of your body turning fat into *ketones* in the liver, can actually infuse the brain with greater energy levels? That's right, and that's just the start. *Ketones* are precious.

Reducing carbohydrates down to the bare minimum begins the process we call ketosis, where the body starts using fat instead of carbs, for its energy source, ergo, its daily fuel. It happens because the body can't find the carbs. *What?! It yells. Where are the damn carbs?* The thing you have been feeding your body for so long and so many years that your body is used to having around is significantly reduced, and so the body has to search for other energy sources, and so it turns to fat, the closest one it can find. Now, what are the benefits of your body processing fat for its energy source rather than carbs?

To begin with, there are a host of products still available when using this diet, including; *eggs, chicken, turkey, tomatoes, spring onions, mushrooms, avocado, bacon, tuna, rocket, many different salads, spices and herbs, salt and pepper, oils such as olive oil, cream, cream cheese, cheddar cheese, mozzarella, many greens including broccoli and asparagus, garlic, and peppers.* Your meals as described in this book will largely consist of these foods. But, onto the benefits of consuming only foods such as these;

Well, the first and most obvious benefit is weight loss. Remove the carbs, and the body works on fat, using it for a productive purpose and hence, burning it off. As a purely weight loss motivated diet, the keto method should start working within *one week*. As you may be aware, it is a highly popular weight loss method, and has worked for many. The process kicks in after only three to four days of consuming 50g or less carbohydrates per day. To put it into perspective, this figure equates to two small bananas, or about three slices of bread, or a single yoghurt.

Further to the weight loss aspect, as it is likely a common reason for taking up the keto diet. First, we will start with fasting, and why we advise against it, and instead, suggest the keto diet. First and foremost, a question. Did you know that fasting can be good for you?

In what way? To what benefit? And how does that relate to ketosis?

Allow me to regale you.

When we fast, the parts of the body that deal with digesting meals (and this is a complex arrangement) stop focusing on this. And what happens then? Well, the body directs its attention elsewhere. Similar to how fasting can encourage this kind of biological development, ketosis also can. Furthermore, fasting is another proven way to kick start the ketosis process. Again, when we fast, our bodies stop focusing on the digesting and processing of food and get to work on other things, and this redirected focus can lead to the body doing some amazing things, some of which have even been attributed to providing health benefits for people with cancer and liver disease, and other debilitating illnesses such as these, but don't quote me on that. There are studies out there, and they are debatably similar kinds of studies to the *ones* that point to ketosis as a proven way of providing benefits in conditions such as heart disease, alzheimers, epilepsy, and parkinson's, amongst many others, which we will briefly look at for some perspective. However, why go to the stress and angst of fasting, when you can simply remove one aspect of your nutritional input, rather than *all* of it at once? Surely, doing so is a much more pleasant experience? Removing the majority of your carbohydrate intake can cause similar reactions in the body in any case.

To anyone still considering the fasting option, I'll put it in the simplest and most appealing way possible. Why fast when you can explore *so many* new and delicious alternatives that are sure to tantalise the taste buds and refresh your palate to an enormous and satisfying degree?

The recipes in this book contain not only *replacements* to your favourite carbohydrates but even *alternatives*. Onions, for instance. Would you realise on first glance that onions are full of sugars that you would want to avoid? Well, there exists such a thing as a spring onion, which will see you through those onion cravings (and they come, believe us), it's how we replace and revitalise the ingredients that count.

Now, there are four different forms of the diet, but bear in mind that only two of these are extensively studied. Also bear in mind that different forms apply to different goals. So examine your goals, and examine our delineations of the forms, and choose which is best for you.

1) **Standard:**

I suppose it's appropriate that we begin with the most highly studied version of the diet - the standard ketogenic diet, which is also the most recommended. This involves a strict low carb intake, a middling protein consumption and high fat diet. In a nutshell, on this diet, it is recommended that carbs make up only ten percent of your sustenance intake. Again, we must stress how this is the most recommended version of the diet, as the cyclical diet and the targeted diet are both targeted towards bodybuilders and those attempting to get gains, and furthermore, the standard diet has been examined and studied the most.

2) **Cyclical:**

This form is when one cuts out carbs completely for five days of the week, and then has a 'carb boost' on the final two days of the week. This sudden high carb intake is often referred to as a 'refeeding' day, and is purported by many to be the better option for attaining muscle gain, and is even claimed to be superior to the standard option. However, please note that little research has been done into the benefits of this, and that the aforementioned comments are purported by those who have been on the diet, and not health experts. However, I will myself purport that there is something to be said for this method. Make no mistake, *carbohydrates are not evil*, and the body fundamentally needs them. Cutting them down in the ketogenic diet is a *short term* change. Long term wise, you need to switch back to carbohydrate intake.

3) **Targeted:**

This is very similar to the standard keto diet, but with some wiggle room. Please note that it is advisable to have been on the standard ketogenic diet for at least 60 days before transitioning over to the targeted version. Why? Well, in layman's terms it is because your body needs to get used to living off of fat. In the initial transition from high carb lifestyles to low carb diets, a keto striving individual often experiences bad side effects at first, such as headaches, fatigue, brain fog, irritability, constipation, insomnia, nausea, dizziness, stomachaches, sugar cravings, cramps, muscle soreness and even something known as *keto breath*, which is simply bad breath caused by the change in intake. Ew. The reason for these side effects is simple. The body is adjusting to a rapid change in lifestyle. And in the case of the targeted diet, the body needs to know how to use glucose while *still* producing those wonderful ketones. At any rate, once you make the switch, the idea is to retain a certain amount of your carbs, which allows for 10 to 15% more carbs than the standard version. Again, *this* is primarily used for bulking and weight gain, so those who are doing this for the gains, and the workouts, this is a possible option for you. But don't jump right in. Again, we stress that the standard diet must be followed for at least 60 days before you make the switch.

4) **High protein:**

Finally, this is similar to the standard plan except with a higher intake of protein. Again, a great option for those who want to lose weight and start to build visible muscles. Protein is one of the key builders of muscle, after all, and equally, protein is tasty. Once you remove carbs, it is great to have another thing to consume in bulk, for the purpose of bulking.

Now, with all that said, let's talk about the major benefits of the diet/lifestyle.

As you may surely be aware, there have been a great many purported benefits to the diet, some even going as far as to claim that it helps with major illnesses such as heart disease, alzheimers, epilepsy and parkinson's. There are even studies which attest to this. For instance, some studies point to the theory that certain types of cancers are helped by it. Some doctors may even recommend the diet alongside chemotherapy, depending on your health situation. This is because the diet causes more oxidative stress in cancer cells, which can cause the cancer cells to die. This, granted, is for certain types of cancer, but still, the idea that a simple change in diet, and it is reasonably simple to switch, can have such power accompanying treatments such as chemotherapy or radiation therapy equally, is an amazing idea. However, it is important to stress that many more future studies need to happen before scientists can affirm with any absolute concrete solidarity that the diet helps to this degree, but still, the mere *suggestion* that it could be that powerful is a true testament to its potential for positive impact.

Another discussion that, even more so than the insulin/glucose argument, can be ascertained with a high probability, is the reduction of cholesterol by consuming certain fats. Of course, healthy fats are always going to be the greater option, e.g avocados, which are extremely high in healthy fats, so much so that apparently about 77% of their calories come from them. High cholesterol is well known as a leading risk riser of cardiovascular disease, and so, the simple act of reducing our cholesterol will reduce that risk. And so, yes, the keto diet can be assumed to be good for this purpose also.

There are even studies to support the notion that a keto diet can help to support our neurological function. This is plausible, due to how the food we consume is a huge benefactor to our mental health. For instance, I am a person who gets depressed when they do not eat much. Furthermore, for many of us, when we are hungry, our mental health issues can worsen. The lack of vitamins will serve to worsen our moods, motivations and tendencies. Were we to then consume healthy foods such as salads, avocados and chicken, onions, tomatoes peppers and mushrooms, our brain chemistry is miraculously and swiftly improved, due to the vitamins directly adding goodness to our brain chemistry. This is a testament to the old adage of *you are what you eat*, except on a mental level. It implies the power of a good diet, and the power of food as a whole. It is important. So don't fast, people.

So what can the keto diet do for our mental health?

A 2019 study supports the notion of improvement in Alzheimer's patients. It does so by analysing the effects of ketosis on ageing brain cells. Equally, a different 2019 study suggests that it can improve the condition of epilepsy. Such are the studies that support the potential benefits of the diet. Quite a list. However, if we are to outline the purported benefits, it is equally germane to highlight some of the risks, which are important to be aware of when undertaking this diet.

It is germane, *mandatory* even, to highlight at this stage that if you have certain conditions, doctors would emphatically not recommend the diet. For instance, those of you who have health conditions of the pancreas, liver, thyroid and gallbladder are not going to be assured of their safety on this diet. This is why it is important that we stress with the utmost sincerity and insistence that you do your research, i.e understand your body, know the risks and if necessary, *check with a medical professional* before undertaking this diet. Because keeping you safe and aware is a priority here. Furthermore, I will outline some further risks, as I believe they are important to mark down for posterity.

For a list of reasons, it is advisable to use the ketogenic diet for *short term purposes*. That is, it should be adhered to for three to six months max. Why? Well, simply put, because it is not advisable as a permanent dietary habit. For instance, there are reports that long term ketogenic dieting can cause *kidney stones*. Research has shown that 13 out of 195 children on the keto diet (as a partial treatment for their epilepsy) developed kidney stones. That seems like a low ratio, but that's 6.6%. Now, for every study claiming that keto causes kidney stones, there is one that claims that the diet is not harmful to the kidneys, and so again, be aware before undertaking this diet!

Moreover, another reported health issue as a result of long term keto dieting is excess protein in the blood. This is logical, seeing as the protein intake here can be relatively high, especially for those choosing the *high protein* option. This condition is characterised by symptoms such as intestinal discomfort and indigestion, dehydration, exhaustion, nausea, irritability, headaches, and/or diarrhea. Another common (and frankly, logical) one is a build up of fat in the

retain more glucose and blood sugar than before. Could this lifestyle be the smoking gun? That said, it is also reported that those on diabetes medication, when they transition to the keto diet, may have to change their meds. So again, make sure you consult your doctor beforehand to figure out all of the kinks!

Moreover, even though risks exist, benefits do too. If the diet is right for you, then look no further than this book, because from here on out there is nothing but delicious recipe after delicious recipe, and if nothing else, the ketogenic diet is certain to make you feel good, lose weight (if that is your aim) and/or gain muscle by a more cleansing means. With certainty, we can say that the ketogenic diet will show results very fast, while recalibrating your dietary habits.

Because although for now, your aim might be to cut the carbs down, the trick lies in how you approach meal times when you *return* to them. Which ones are healthy? Which ones should you avoid? Now that the carbs have been out of your system for the last three to six months, the cravings are likely to be gone as well, due to the fact that you have removed them, which should give you the wonderful advantage of being able to approach carbohydrates *objectively*, with reason, and with much more awareness than before. Knowledge is power, and so is the process of abstaining, changing things up, and enjoying a radically different lifestyle for a while.

(*Please note that on certain recipes, particularly the Side Dishes *segment, the carbohydrate intake is higher than the recommended max. This is because all of the nutritional information is in total, rather than per serving. For per serving, please note the number each meal serves, as is noted on certain recipes where carb level is higher than the recommended max*)*

Breakfast

As the old adage goes, breakfast should be the most important meal of the day. It fuels us when we are travelling to work, walking our dogs, or going to the gym, and should keep us energised throughout the entirety of the day. Where would we be without it? Think of all the days in your life where you have begun with a hearty breakfast, and all the days you have not, and consider, which were better? On which days did you have the most energy? The answer of course is the days where you had breakfast. It lined your stomach with the goods to keep you happy, healthy and energised. And so, these carefully considered recipes are designed to energise you to the max. They are chock full of a great deal of nutritional goodness in them, as well as being tasty. The ultimate combo. Wakey wakey. But where do we start? And how on earth does one attain breakfast without the aid, sustenance and crunchy, buttery goodness of our reigning monarch bread, and her royal king butter, or the carbohydrates in our favourite cereals? Well, it just so happens that such a thing as keto-friendly bread exists, and you'll see it in some of these recipes. But, thank God, eggs are still an option, right? What can we do without bread? Some interesting things, let me tell you, and not all of them involve eggs, I promise. Below, you will find a range of meals ranging in sizes and proportions. The first thing that you will realise when taking your first look at ketogenic sustenance options is that there are plenty of energising foods that will carry you through to your lunch hour with some to spare as well. Not only are these meals nutritious, but some of them contain more energy within them than your standard breakfasts of bacon sandwiches or cereal. So leaf on through and see what you like the look of. May I heartily recommend the cinnamon waffle? Sorry, that was my sweet tooth talking. Enjoy.

Bacon & Eggs With Mushrooms

High in protein and *high* in fat

CALORIES (KCAL): 435 | CARBS: 2.2G | PROTEIN: 34G | FAT: 33G

SERVES: 2 ADULTS

INGREDIENTS:

○ 4 x large eggs

○ 1 - 2 x cups mushrooms

○ 4 x slices bacon

○ 6 - 8 x cherry tomatoes

○ ½ tsp ground black pepper

○ ½ tbsp olive oil

○ ½ x cup fresh thyme

○ ½ x cup fresh asparagus

○ ½ x tbsp butter

METHOD:

1 Cook the bacon in a pan, oven or grill until medium to crispy. Once done, leave in the oven to keep warm.

2 Line a pan with butter and fry the eggs on a medium heat (if you choose to cook your bacon in a pan, use the same pan, utilising the bacon gristle as ballast). You can also use a measuring jug here to avoid spillage. If sunny side up is your tipple, leave the eggs to cook without flipping. Otherwise, flip them carefully and cook them for an extra 90 seconds.

3 Chop the cherry tomatoes and mushrooms in half, and the fresh asparagus into thin slices. Fry in a separate pan, simultaneously with the bacon and eggs.

4 Assemble the meal. Sprinkle your salt and ground black pepper on the egg yolks and bacon to add to the taste, as well as adding the fresh thyme. Add the vegetables and enjoy!

Fried Eggs & Greens

Moderate in protein and *moderate* in fat
**CALORIES (KCAL): 156 CAL | CARBS: 1.2G | PROTEIN: 12G | FAT: 10G
SERVES: 1 - 2 ADULTS**

INGREDIENTS:

○ 2 x eggs

○ 1 x tbsp of olive oil

○ 2 x tbsp butter

○ 1 x tsp black pepper

○ 1 x avocado

○ 1 x cup fine sliced broccoli

○ ½ x cup spinach

○ ½ x red spring onion

METHOD:

1   Melt the butter in the pan, and crack on with the eggs, and get them going on a medium heat. Cook for 8-10 minutes.

2   Pour the oil in a separate pan, chop the broccoli and spinach, and add them to the pan. Heat until sizzling and stir. Cook for 8-10 minutes and then serve.

3   Slice the avocado into eight segments and add to the bed of greens. Chop and dice the red spring onion. Add.

4   Remove the eggs from the pan and sprinkle them with the black pepper, and serve.

Avocado and Bacon Bagel

High in protein and ***moderate*** in fat
CALORIES (KCAL): 400 | CARBS: 15G | PROTEIN: 40G | FAT: 15G
SERVES: 1 - 2 ADULTS

INGREDIENTS:

○ 1 x avocado

○ 1 x low carb bagel

○ 2 x bacon slices

○ 1 x tomato

○ ½ x red spring onion

○ 1 x cup coriander

○ 1 x tsp olive oil

METHOD:

1   Put the oil in a pan, put on a medium heat. Add bacon, turning occasionally. Cook until satisfied.

2   Take your low carb bagel and slice and toast until satisfied.

3   Chop the red spring onion as well as the tomato and coriander, and blend all three ingredients together to make pico.

4   Plate up the bagel. Slice and smash the avocado, take out the stone, and smash the avocado over each slice of the bagel half and half.

5   Sprinkle the pico over the avocado bagel slices, place bacon over the top. Serve and enjoy.

Deviled Eggs

High in protein and *high* in fat
CALORIES (KCAL): 936 CALORIES (TOTAL) | CARBS: 7.2G | PROTEIN: 72G | FAT: 60G
SERVES: 4 - 6 ADULTS

INGREDIENTS:

○ 12 x eggs (make sure these are not fridge temperature, as they will boil better if room temperature)

○ 1 x cup cream cheese (softened by room temperature)

○ ½ x tsp salt

○ 1 x grind black pepper

○ 2 x tbsp bagel seasoning

○ Red pepper flakes

METHOD:

1 Hard boil the eggs in a way of your preference (the most efficient is to bring a pan to a boil and lower the eggs in. Simmer for 10 minutes to achieve a hard boil) then drain the eggs, and cool them. Peel.

2 Cut the eggs in half and throw the yolks into a separate bowl. Slice the cream cheese into pieces, add and blend with the yolks. Add salt and pepper. Beat until soft and fluffy. Add red pepper flakes.

3 Spoon the yolk mixture into the egg whites. If stiff or hard, microwave for 1-4 seconds to soften.

4 Sprinkle the yolky egg whites with bagel seasoning.

Cinnamon Waffle

Moderate in protein and *moderate* in fat
CALORIES (KCAL): 293 | CARBS: 5G | PROTEIN: 13.8 | FAT: 23.3G
SERVES: 1 - 2 ADULTS

INGREDIENTS:

○ 2 x eggs

○ 1 x tbsp erythritol (or your preferred sugar substitute)

○ 5 x tbsp almond flour

○ 2 x tsp vanilla extract (in total, it is used multiple times)

○ ¼x tsp bicarbonate of soda

○ 2 x tbsp cream cheese

○ 1 x tbsp double cream

○ ¼ x tsp cinnamon

METHOD:

1 Break the first egg into a bowl and add erythritol and mix. Add almond flour, mix until it is a dark golden brown colour and there are no lumps. Add a second egg and continue to mix until the batter is smooth. Pour into the waffle maker and heat up.

2 Add the cream cheese to a separate bowl, adding the double cream and cinnamon and some of the batter (reserve some of the batter for this purpose) plus, add the ¼ tsp of the vanilla extract. Mix well.

3 Serve waffles when cooked, add filling and serve.

Bacon and Broccoli Burrito with Peppers and Cheese

Moderate in protein and *moderate* in fat

CALORIES (KCAL): 259 | CARBS: 9.69G | PROTEIN: 13.8 | FAT: 18.4G
SERVES: 1 - 2 ADULTS

INGREDIENTS:

○ 2 x bacon slices

○ 1 x cup chopped broccoli

○ 1 x chopped tomato

○ 2 x large eggs

○ 1 tbsp low carb milk

○ ½ x cup of red peppers

○ ½ x cup of green peppers

○ 1 x spring onion

- ○ ¼ tsp table salt

- ○ ¼ tsp ground black pepper

- ○ 2 tbsp grated cheese

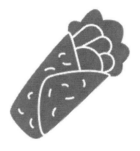

METHOD:

1. Cook the bacon on a medium heat, regularly turning for 6 - 8 minutes until the bacon is crisp. Remove the bacon from the pan and add broccoli. Cook for 3 - 4 minutes until soft and then cut and add the tomato. Chop peppers and add them too. Stir in for 2 - 3 minutes and then transfer to a separate bowl.

2. Slice up the spring onion, whisk the eggs with milk. Add the pepper and salt. Continue mixing.

3. Add oil to your vegetable pan and pour the egg mixture carefully in. Cook on a steady, medium heat until the bottom sets like an omelette (2 - 3 minutes). Carefully flip using a thin, wide spatula, lather with cheese and continue cooking on a steady medium heat until it sets entirely.

4. Fill the burrito with bacon and broccoli (as befits your style and taste) and roll up into a classic burrito.

5. Serve and enjoy!

Sausage Keto Club Sandwich

Moderate in protein and *high* in fat
**CALORIES (KCAL): 602 | CARBS: 7.2G | PROTEIN: 24G | FAT: 54G
SERVES: 1 - 2 - 3 ADULTS (AS NEEDED)**

INGREDIENTS:

○ 4 x sausages

○ 2 x eggs

○ 2 x tbsp cream cheese

○ 4 x tbsp cheddar cheese

○ 1 x avocado, sliced

○ 1 tsp paprika

○ ¼ tsp table salt

○ 1/ 4 tsp ground black pepper

○ 2 x tomatoes, wheel sliced

○ 2 x cups rocket salad

○ 2 - 6 x slices ketogenic bread (as needed)

METHOD:

1   Cook the sausages on a medium heat (as per the packet branding instructions). Cook until done and then place on a plate.

2   Put the cream cheese and cheddar cheese into a separate bowl and microwave until soft (30 - 35 seconds) and then mix in salt, paprika and ground black pepper into the bowl, whisk until mixed.

3   Whisk the eggs and then cook on a steady, medium heat. Add the cheese and seasoning (cheesoning?) with the eggs and cook until set, into an omelette. Flip and slice.

4   Slice the avocados thinly and lay over keto friendly bread, with rocket salad. Slice the sausages, lay them over the avocado and rocket, add the omelette mix to each sandwich. Assemble carefully.

5   Serve and smile.

Scrambled Eggs With Pepperoni and Guacamole

Moderate in protein and *high* in fat

CALORIES (KCAL): 450 | CARBS: 1.5G | PROTEIN: 26G | FAT: 40G
SERVES: 1 - 2 ADULTS

INGREDIENTS:

○ 3 x large eggs

○ 1 x tbsp cream cheese (optional)

○ 1 x tsp salt

○ 1 x tsp ground black pepper

○ 1 ½ x cups pepperoni

○ ½ x red spring onion

○ 3 x cherry tomatoes

○ 1 x tbsp butter

- ⭘ 1 x cup grated cheddar cheese

- ⭘ 1 x tbsp salsa

- ⭘ 1 x avocado

- ⭘ 1 x lime

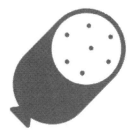

METHOD:

1. Break the eggs into a bowl and whisk. Add the pepperoni and the cream cheese and mix. Add tomatoes (reserving some for later) and ground black pepper, and continue mixing. Add salt.

2. Melt the butter in a pan and add the pepperoni and egg mixture. Stir on a medium heat until the eggs start to scramble. Continue stirring until done and then plate it up. Add grated cheddar cheese, salsa, and salad.

3. Cut open the avocado, half it and smash it. Add it to a separate bowl, adding also the reserved tomatoes, chopped red spring onion, and squeeze the lime over it, mixing carefully. Add a pinch of salt. Add to the plate.

Avocado Egg Cakes with Bacon Salutes

Moderate in protein and *moderate* in fat

CALORIES (KCAL): 412 | CARBS: 2.2G | PROTEIN: 25G | FAT: 35G
SERVES: 1 - 2 ADULTS

INGREDIENTS:

○ 2 - 4 x large eggs (as needed)

○ 2 - 4 x slices bacon (as needed)

○ 2 x avocados

○ 1 x tbsp olive oil

○ 2 x tbsp table salt

○ ½ x black ground pepper

○ ½ x cup green jalapenos (optional)

METHOD:

1 Fill a pan with water and set to boil on a high heat. Place the eggs in, making sure they are submerged by at least 1 inch. Cover the pan, and bring the water to a boil. Once boiling steadily, take the pan off of the hob, and rest the eggs for 10 - 15 minutes. Place in a colander and run them beneath a tap until cooled and then peel.

2 Lay a sheet of aluminium foil over a baking tray and place your bacon slices on the tray. Place in the middle of a preheated oven, on the middle shelf. Cook the bacon until done and then take it out of the oven, leaving it to cool. Once this is achieved, snip the bacon into triangular shapes, or small falkes, as preferred.

3 Line a small, separate pan with ketogenic cooking oil and turn the dial to a medium heat. Chop your green jalapenos into small pieces, place them in the pan. Heat until sizzling, cook until they are good and fried and then remove.

4 Slice the eggs in half vertically, carefully remove the yolks and place them in a bowl. Half and peel the avocados, place in a bowl with the yolks, add the olive oil, salt and ground black pepper, and mash the mixture together. Add the green jalapenos last.

5 For the assembly stage, scoop the yolk, avocado, oil and jalapeno mix into the egg whites, inserting the bacon last to salute you for the day.

Mushroom Burrito with Sausages and Greens

High in protein and *high* in fat

CALORIES (KCAL): 626 | CARBS: 5.9 | PROTEIN: 53.8 | FAT: 77.8G
SERVES: 1 - 2 ADULTS (ADJUST INGREDIENTS AS NEEDED)

INGREDIENTS:

○ 2 - 4 x sausages (as needed)

○ 1 - 2 x cups mushrooms (as needed)

○ 2 x large eggs

○ 1 x tbsp cream cheese

○ 1 x tbsp low carb milk

○ 1 x cup asparagus

○ ½ x cup green peppers

○ ½ x cup broccoli

○ 1 x tbsp olive oil

○ 1 x tsp full fat butter

○ 1 x tsp ground black pepper

○ 1 x tsp table salt

METHOD:

1   Place the sausages under the grill on a medium heat. Cook until ready (as per packaging instructions)

2   Chop up the asparagus, green peppers and broccoli into tiny pieces and merge together. Line a small pan with olive oil, place the vegetables in the pan and cook on a medium to high heat, stirring occasionally.

3   Break the large eggs into a mixing jug, adding the cream, milk, black pepper and salt to taste. Whisk the ingredients together until they are appropriately mixed.

4   Pour the egg mixture carefully into the vegetable pan and cook on a steady and consistent heat (medium heat) until the bottom sets (2 - 3 minutes) and then flip using a thin, wide spatula. Sprinkle the cheese over it and then continue cooking until it sets entirely.

5   Plate up the burrito and greens, add the sausages. Serve and enjoy.

Lunch

It's approaching that hour. Lunch time is coming. Not the most important meal of the day, but it's certainly the one that carries us through the afternoon and sees us home. Unlike breakfast, which demands speed and efficiency, due to our societal need to eat and go in the morning, lunch is something of a different beast. Lunch is something we carry around with us. To work, or college or the gym, or university. Lunch is something that demands simplicity, and convenience. Dare I say, when we are almost ready to wave the white flag in the midst of our day, lunch comes at us like a shining silver milestone, ready to give us that extra ballast to hurtle us forward to the end of our day. To, as we will explore later, dinner time. But what on earth can we do that is tasty, filling and keto friendly? One thing you may notice about some of these meals is that they are transferable to other meal times. A tuna salad, for instance, which we will look at in a ketogenic method in just a second, is easily transferable. The meal laid out below is a simple formula, but the mere application of, say, avocados or even eggs can turn this meal into something more substantial, that is also chock full of nutrients, and terrific energy sources. But for the purposes of this recipe, we'll just say that many of these meals can be done in much simpler ways, it is those extra doses of seasoning, pepper and whatnot that make them all the more tasty and delicious, and so yes, regardless of the ingredients, there are a great many dishes we can assemble relatively easily, without having to change a heck of a lot of our cupboard and fridge contents. The ones we shall delineate will contain a range of nutritional variety, ranging from moderate protein to high fat. One thing they all have in common though, is a low intake of carbohydrates. Best of all though, is their convenience!

A Classic Keto Simple Tuna Salad

Moderate in protein and *moderate* in fat

CALORIES (KCAL): 642 | CARBS: 17.2 | PROTEIN: 32.2G | FAT: 50.3G
SERVES: 1 - 2 ADULTS

INGREDIENTS

○ 1 x tin tuna

○ 4 x celery sticks

○ 1 x cups quartered cherry tomatoes

○ 1 x cup salad of your choice

○ ½ x cucumber

○ 2 x tbsp mayonnaise

○ 1 x avocado

○ 1/4 x cups mushrooms

○ 1 x cups asparagus

METHOD:

1 Open and drain the tuna and place in a bowl. Add the mayonnaise and mix appropriately.

2 Chop the celery into segments of your preference, and slice the tomato into larger segments, four or eight, depending on how many tomatoes you want to use. Chop and lay out your cucumber, asparagus, ketogenic salad leaves, and mushrooms; creating a crunchy, crispy bed of greens. Peel your avocado, remove the stone and slice it into 8 segments using a serrated knife, nudge them out and then place them around the salad.

3 Mix the tuna mayo at your favourite ratio and then smooth it over your greens, and eat.

Mushroom and Tomato Omelette with Ham

High in protein and *high* in fat

CALORIES (KCAL): 565 | CARBS: 3.5 | PROTEIN: 51G | FAT: 59G

SERVES: 1 - 2 ADULTS

INGREDIENTS:

○ 3 x large eggs

○ 1 x cups mushrooms

○ 2 x diced tomatoes

○ 4 x quartered cherry tomatoes

○ 3 x tbsp cheddar cheese

○ 1 x cup ketogenic salad of you choice

○ 1 x tbsp green pesto

○ 1 x tbsp olive oil

○ ½ x cups of ham (not honey glazed)

○ 1 x tsp ground black pepper

○ 1 x tsp salt

METHOD:

1 Crack the eggs into a bowl, whisk them until smooth, adding salt. Grate your cheese (make sure you use an unprocessed cheese such as cheddar cheese or mozzarella) and add some to the egg mixture. Melt the oil in a large frying pan until it starts to sizzle away, and then pour the egg mixture in.

2 Chop and dice the mushrooms and tomatoes (sparing one or two for the salad), and snip your ham into small bits with a pair of kitchen shears.

3 Carefully add a layer of cheese to the pan-bound egg mixture, followed by mushrooms (these take the longest to cook) then the ham, tomatoes, followed by a second layer of cheese. Let the ingredients slowly cook and fuse together, turning golden brown and delicious, adding black pepper to taste. Take one to two teaspoons full of green pesto and smooth it over the surface of the omelette.

4 Now that the mixture is in the pan, turn the heat down and cook slowly on a low heat for about 15 minutes. Assemble the salad, adding the quartered tomatoes, and then finally, the finished omelette. Enjoy!

Sauteed Rocket with Mushrooms

Moderate in protein and *moderate - high* in fat
CALORIES (KCAL): 666.1 | CARBS: 4.7G | PROTEIN: 27.5G | FAT: 61.3G
SERVES: 1 ADULTS

INGREDIENTS:

○ 1 x cups mushrooms

○ 2 x tbsp olive oil

○ 8 x cups rocket salad

○ 1 x spring onion, sliced

○ 4 x ground garlic cloves

○ ½ x tsp salt

○ 28g red pepper flakes

○ 4 x tbsp grated cheddar cheese

METHOD:

1 Chop the mushrooms into quarters, slice the red spring onion and grind the garlic cloves. Using a large pan, add olive oil to its surface, heat up and then add all of the above vegetables and garlic.

2 Stir until vegetables start to shrink, and the mushrooms begin to ooze. Add the red pepper flakes, salt, rocket, and cheddar cheese. Stir and mix.

3 Serve and enjoy.

Classic Keto Peppery Chicken Stir Fried Salad

Moderate-high in protein and *low* in fat
CALORIES (KCAL): 180 | CARBS: 0G | PROTEIN: 41G | FAT: 1.9G
SERVES: 2 - 4 ADULTS

INGREDIENTS:

O 2 x chicken breasts

O 8 x cups rocket salad

O 1 x red pepper

O 1 x green pepper

O 1 x yellow pepper

O ½ x cucumber

O 1 x garlic and herb dressing

O 1 x tomato, sliced

O 1 x spring onion, diced

O 1 x avocado

O 4 x ground garlic cloves

O 2 x tbsp olive oil

METHOD:

1 Preheat the oven and line a baking tray with aluminium foil, covering it in a reasonable amount of olive oil (so the chicken doesn't stick to the tray). Place the chicken breasts on the tray and insert the tray into the oven on the middle shelf. Cook on a medium heat until done (20 - 30 minutes).

2 Chop up the green pepper, red pepper and yellow pepper, and spring spring onions. Dice the cucumber and the red spring onion. Drizzle some olive oil in a large pan and turn the hob dial to a medium heat. Place the vegetables into the pan, stirring until they begin to sizzle and fry. Continue stirring until the spring onions start to go crispy brown, and then add the arugula (rocket salad). Continue stirring on a lower heat.

3 Once the chicken is cooked, remove it from the oven and place it to the side. Wait until it has cooled (to a level manageable to handle), remove it from the tray and place it on an appropriate chopping board and slice into either long slices, or a small, diced size (as preferred) and then add to the vegetable pan.

4 Plate up, adding the garlic and herb dressing.

Smoked Salmon and Greens

Moderate - low in protein and *moderate - low* in fat

CALORIES (KCAL): 468.8 | CARBS: 10G | PROTEIN: 28G | FAT: 23.1G
SERVES: 2 ADULTS

INGREDIENTS:

- ○ 2 x 1 serving size salmon fillets

- ○ 1 x cups asparagus

- ○ 1 x cups broccoli

- ○ 1 x cups ketogenic salad of your choice

- ○ 4 x ground garlic cloves

- ○ 2 x tbsp chopped parsley

- ○ 4 x tbsp grated parmesan cheese

- ○ 2 tbsp olive oil

- ○ 1 x tbsp ground black pepper

METHOD:

1 Take your small salmon fillets and remove the skin. Preheat the oven to medium heat, take a baking tray and line it with aluminium foil. Season the salmon fillets with salt and pepper and place them on the tray.

2 Mix the butter in a moderate sized bowl with the parmesan cheese and the parsley, and whisk these ingredients together. Grind the garlic cloves and add half of them to this mix, continue mixing, reserving the other half of the garlic for the greens.

3 Cover the salmon in the mixture, and then place the relay in the centre of the oven, cooking for approximately 20 - 25 minutes until golden coloured. Once they are cooked through, flip them over and continue cooking for an additional 4 - 5 minutes so that they are completely cooked.

4 Simultaneously to this, chop the asparagus and the broccoli. Take a small pan and line it with olive oil, place the greens in the pan and cook steadily for 10 - 15 minutes until sauteed.

5 Remove the greens from the pan and place on plates, remove also the salmon from the oven and place these on the plates as well. You are now done. Enjoy!

Classic Keto Chicken Salad

High in protein and ***Moderate*** in fat
CALORIES (KCAL): 730 | CARBS: 17.3 | PROTEIN: 111.3G | FAT: 66.2G
SERVES: 1 - 2 ADULTS

INGREDIENTS:

○ 2 x tbsp olive oil

○ 2 x chicken breast fillets

○ 1 x avocado

○ ½ x red pepper

○ 3 x tbsp coriander

○ 1 x ground black pepper

○ 1 x tsp salt (to taste)

○ 1 x tsp cayenne

○ 3 x tbsp mayonnaise

○ 1 x tbsp lime juice

○ 2 x tbsp balsamic vinegar

○ 1 x lemon

METHOD:

1   Drizzle a tbsp of olive oil into a medium sized pan. Lay the chicken breasts in the pan and cook on a medium heat. Cook until the chicken is cooked fully through, turning occasionally. Once done, remove from the pan and place in a bowl (to avoid spillage). Leave it to cool and then shred it using a knife and fork or two forks.

2   Cut the avocado in half, remove the stone, and then slice into wedges or cubes. Take the red pepper and slice it in half, dicing it. Finally, chop the coriander, and then add all ingredients in with the chicken. Add the pepper, salt, cayenne and lime juice and then mix the salad together, topping it off with a drizzle of balsamic vinegar and a lemon.

Classic Keto Turkey Salad

Moderate in protein and *low* in fat

CALORIES (KCAL): 189 | CARBS: 0.1G | PROTEIN: 30G | FAT: 7G
SERVES: 1 - 2 ADULTS

INGREDIENTS:

○ 1 x tbsp erythritol

○ ½ x spring onion, thinly sliced

○ ½ x tsp ground black pepper

○ 2 x celery sticks

○ 1 x tbsp olive oil

○ 2 x turkey breast steaks

○ 1 x tbsp coriander

○ 2 x tbsp mayonnaise

○ ½ x yellow pepper

METHOD:

1. Use a medium sized pan. Place a tbsp olive oil in the pan and turn the hob dial up to a medium heat. Take the turkey steaks and place them in the pan, and cook for about 4 minutes, turn, and cook for an additional 4 minutes. Once cooked, dispense them from the pan into a bowl. Using two forks, pull the turkey apart into shredded pieces.

2. Chop the celery sticks, yellow pepper, spring onion, and the coriander, and place them in the bowl with the shredded turkey steaks. Add the tbsp of mayonnaise, the ground black pepper, the tsp of salt and the tbsp of erythritol. Mix the ingredients all together and serve.

Bunless Beef Burgers with Sauteed Vegetable Salad

Moderate in protein and *moderate-high* in fat
**CALORIES (KCAL): 725 | CARBS: 13.9G | PROTEIN: 48.4 | FAT: 62.6G
SERVES: 1 ADULT**

INGREDIENTS:

○ 2 x beef burger patties

○ 1 x cup arugula

○ 2 x tbsp olive oil

○ 2 x tomatoes

○ ½ x red pepper

○ 1 x cup mushrooms

○ 3 x ground garlic cloves

○ 1 x ground black pepper

○ ¼ tsp salt (to taste)

METHOD:

1 Using a medium sized pan, place a tbsp of olive oil in the middle of the pan, spread around and turn the hob on a medium heat. Place the beef burgers in the pan and cook steadily, cooking on both slides for roughly 3 minutes on each side.

2 Chop the mushrooms, pepper and tomatoes. Grind the garlic cloves. Using a separate pan, place another tbsp of olive oil in the pan, heat on medium and add the vegetables and arugula. Cook for 10 minutes or so until the flavours blend together, adding the salt and pepper.

3 Remove the burgers and plate them up. Remove the sauteed vegetables and place them on the plate with the burgers.

4 Enjoy!

Main Dishes

If breakfast is the most important meal of the day, then dinner is surely the second most important? It stands to reason, does it not? If the purpose of breakfast is to boost us up for the day, and give us a well needed lining of strength in our bellies which we use to soldier through what awaits us, both in a physical sense, but rather equally importantly, in a mental capacity, then this meal time allows for lunch time to be a smaller affair, does it not? Sandwiches, salads, small omelettes, jacket potatoes (or more appropriately, the substitutes that we have delineated in the previous section) are what we consider, generally, as lunch time meals. Much smaller dishes than the typical idea of a substantial breakfast, as our previous meal. And so, would it do to have a small dinner after a small lunch? I think not. Furthermore, if the gap between breakfast and dinner is sustained only by a smaller meal, and our bodies are running off the energy of breakfast for the vast proportion of our busiest hours, then surely dinner time needs to be just as substantial in its own right, for the sake of the evenings. Many of us have busy evenings. It's when we tend to our hobbies, or our children, or our workout regime, and therefore dinner, to put it in a mildly philosophical way, is the breakfast of night time, is it not? That's why, for this portion of the book, we will show you how to whip up poultry meat in as satisfying and healthy a manner as you can imagine. Where we bring out our proverbial big guns. This, ladies and gentlemen, is where it gets really real.

Please note that in this section we will delineate a variety of meals, accounting for a range of different nutritional intake rates. Some will consist of high protein and low fat, while others will lean towards high fat, and to the latter I stress this: high fat is a good thing on the keto diet. Fat is a large supply of your energy. Fat is your juice. Societally, we discriminate against fat. Well, now is the time to discriminate against the discrimination. Fat is your friend.

Ketogenic Chicken Pasta with Pesto

High in protein, ***low*** in fat

CALORIES (KCAL): 465 | CARBS: 14.6 | PROTEIN: 151.4G | FAT: 18.5
SERVES: 1 - 2 - 3 ADULTS (DEPENDING ON PORTIONS)

INGREDIENTS:

○ 1 x packet gluten free pasta

○ 1 x jar green pesto

○ 1 x sliced spring onion

○ 3 x tomatoes sliced

○ 1 ½ cups mushrooms

○ 1 x pepper (red, green, yellow or orange, depending on preference)

○ 2 x chicken breasts

○ 1 x tbsp keto chicken seasoning (of your choice)

○ 4 x celery sticks

○ 3 - 4 x ground garlic cloves

○ 4 x bacon slices

○ 2 x tbsp olive oil

○ ½ x cup coriander (chopped)

METHOD:

1   Preheat the oven for 10 - 15 minutes.

2   Line a baking tray with aluminium foil and douse lightly in olive oil. Place the chicken breasts on the tray and place in the centre of the oven on a medium heat. Cook for 20 - 30 minutes until golden brown.

3   Line a small pan with oil and heat up on a mid - low heat, place the bacon strips in the pan, cooking steadily, turning occasionally with tongs (avoiding splashes). Cook the bacon for 10 - 15 minutes until crispy and then place to the side.

4   Slice and dice your spring onion and tomatoes and peppers, and quarter the mushrooms. Chop the celery sticks into thin, sickle moon shapes and grind the garlic cloves. In a large pan, place more oil, and place the diced spring onion in. Cook until it starts to brown adn then add the tomatoes, peppers, celery sticks and garlic. Stir regularly, making sure all veg gets cooked equally and evenly.

5 Remove the cooked chicken from the oven and place on an appropriate chopping board. Chop into bite sized pieces, and finely chop the bacon (to make that pesto pop!), and add your chicken and bacon to the vegetable pan and continue to stir, cooking evenly.

6 Boil some water in a round, deep pan. Heat until bubbling and popping and then measure and add the gluten free pasta. Cook until al dente and then drain in a colander and add to the vegetable pan. Add green pesto, seasoning, coriander and stir well until well mixed (a good ratio) and piping hot. Serve.

Keto Fish And Chips

High in protein and ***high*** in fat

CALORIES (KCAL): 740 | CARBS: 6.2G | PROTEIN: 43G | FAT: 60G
SERVES: UP TO 4 ADULTS

INGREDIENTS:

○ 4 x fish fillets of your choice

○ 2 x tbsp olive oil

○ 1 x cup ground macadamia nuts

○ 2 x avocados

○ 2 x large eggs

○ 1 x tbsp pouring cream

○ 1 x tsp red chilli flakes (optional, preference determinant)

○ ½ x cup grated cheese (preferably parmesan)

○ ½ x cup chopped parsley

○ 4 x tomatoes (quartered)

○ 1 ½ x cups almond meal

METHOD:

1   Whisk the eggs, cream and a dash of water (to batter) in a large bowl, and in a separate bowl, mix together the cheese, almond meal, parsley and red chilli flakes (if using, this will really spruce up the flavour!)

2   Halve and peel the avocados, remove the stones and chop into (up to) 8 wedges, coating said wedges in egg mixture (individually), and then coating them a second time, in the almond, cheese and parsley mixture. Cover them in oil and place on a baking tray in a preheated oven, on medium heat for 20 - 25 minutes.

3   Repeat the above motion with the fish fillets. Cover the fish fillets in the ground macadamia nuts. Put olive oil in a large pan and heat up. Place the fillets individually in the pan, frying evenly on each side for 2 - 3 minutes on each side. Alternatively you can cook the fillets in an oven on a medium heat at a time of 20 - 25 minutes, with the avocados.

4   Place the cooked fish on a plate, with the avocado chips, and serve with salad, tomatoes and a side of lemon.

Fried Prawns with Cauliflower Rice and Rocket

Moderate in protein and *low* in fat

CALORIES (KCAL): 566 | CARBS: 22.3G | PROTEIN: 35.8G | FAT: 2.8G
SERVES: UP TO 4 ADULTS

INGREDIENTS:

○ 4 x ground garlic cloves

○ 1 x tbsp ground black pepper

○ 1 x tbsp olive oil

○ 1 x tbsp paprika

○ 2 x cups peeled prawns

○ 3 x cups cauliflower rice

○ 1 x tbsp butter

○ 1 x cup milk

○ 1 x cups garlic powder

○ 1 ½ x cups arugula

liver. The liver generally operates with a low level of fat, and a high build up of excess fat can cause health concerns. Simply put, the liver can do without that excess fat, and the keto diet, over a long term, will cause a build up.

The last two I will mention are commonly reported, and related. The first is a mineral and vitamin deficiency, which can cause a plethora of symptoms including an irregular heartbeat and loss of appetite, to name just a couple. Furthermore, *a low tolerance for exercise* is also commonly reported, and a vitamin deficiency is a likely culprit for this. Which is no good for those of us who are turning to the keto diet for body building purposes.

In summary, the keto diet holds a great deal of short term health benefits, and is wonderful for losing weight, but is highly inadvisable to commit to for the long run. Because at the end of the day, although we are cutting carbs down to the minimum of less than 50g per day, never forget that the human body fundamentally *needs* carbohydrates, which is an important thing to remember when going forwards with this diet.

I'd like to assess much of the contrasting studies. It is likely down to the diet being relatively new, and there being so few consolidated studies that can confirm one way or another - however, since the reports of these issues exist, it is important to note them. Please remember that these effects are caused by *long term* keto dieting, and we advise it for the short term of 3 to 6 months, for optimal results, and the ultimate diet recalibration.

So, with that being said, one thing beyond this is true, and that is that ketones are *good for the liver*. So, it stands to reason that the ketogenic diet would help with illnesses such as liver issues. Or hell, another believable idea is that it could help with diabetes. Think about it: when carb intake is severely down, your body burns fat instead of glucose or blood sugar. This means that the body would

METHOD:

1 Peel the prawns. Stir the paprika with the garlic powder in a medium sized bowl. Now, coat the prawns in the mixture and set to the side.

2 Grind the garlic cloves. Heat the olive oil in a medium sized pan on a medium heat, placing the rocket leaves and garlic into the pan, stirring until moist and delicious looking, and then season with salt and black pepper, adding the coated prawns once done and cooking for 5 minutes or so, seasoning again with salt and pepper.

3 Melt the butter in a deep pan, add the cauliflower rice and steadily stir while adding milk to the pan. Keep stirring until the cauliflower rice is rich and creamy, and then add the rest of milk and continue stirring. This should take around 15 - 18 minutes in total.

4 Divide between four and serve!

Chicken Sauce With Low Carb Keto Noodles

Very high in protein and *very high* in fat
CALORIES (KCAL): 1,756 | CARBS: 25.2G | PROTEIN: 121.5G | FAT: 107.8G
SERVES: 4 ADULTS

INGREDIENTS:

○ 1 - 2 x spring onions (diced)

○ 4 x large tomatoes (diced)

○ 1 x cups mushrooms

○ 1 x red pepper

○ 3 x celery sticks

○ 2 x can chopped tomatoes

○ 4 x ground garlic cloves

○ 1 x tbsp ground black pepper

○ 1 x tsp cayenne

○ 1 x tbsp olive oil

○ 1 x tsp oregano

○ 2 x chicken breast fillets

○ 2 x cups shredded cheddar cheese or mozzarella

○ 3 x large eggs

METHOD:

1   Microwave the three cups of cheese, pausing every 40 seconds or so to stir. The process should take 3 minutes max to work. Crack the eggs into a bowl, remove the yolks and mix the yolks with the melted cheese. Mix until the ingredients start to solidify and take shape.

2   Take the mixture - it should be shaped like a ball - and place it on a solid, non-stick surface e.g parchment paper or a wooden chopping board and roll it flat with a rolling pin, and then cut it into the desired noodle shapes, and refrigerate until it solidifies. Warning: This may have to be left overnight to slidify, so make sure you plan this meal ahead).

3   Preheat the oven to around 190 degrees celsius. Line a baking tray with aluminium foil and douse it with olive oil. Place the chicken breast fillets on the tray and cook in the oven for 25 - 30 minutes.

4 Dice the spring onion, peppers and tomatoes and quarter the mushrooms. Grind the garlic cloves and chop the celery sticks. Using a large pan, drizzle olive oil into the centre and put on a medium heat, adding the spring onion and frying until browning. Add the peppers, tomatoes, mushrooms, garlic cloves and celery sticks. Stir until well balanced and mixed.

5 Remove the chicken breast fillets and place to the side. Allow to cool for a moment and then chop and dice into small chicken pieces or strips, depending on preference. Add the chicken to the vegetable mix and continue to stir, adding the two cans of chopped tomatoes. Add the grind of black pepper, the salt, cayenne, and the oregano.

Fried Chicken and Greens

Moderate-low in protein and *Moderate-low* in fat

**CALORIES (KCAL): 1,321 | CARBS: 14.7G | PROTEIN: 36G | FAT: 35.2G
SERVES: 1 - 2 ADULTS**

INGREDIENTS:

- 2 x tbsp olive oil
- 1 x cup broccoli
- 2 - 4 x chicken breast fillets
- 1 tbsp black pepper
- ½ x tsp salt
- 2 x celery sticks
- 1 x cup cauliflower

METHOD:

1   Rinse the broccoli and chop into small, bite sized pieces. Chop the celery sticks into sickle moons.

2   Heat a tbsp of olive oil in a medium sized pan. Place your chicken breast fillets in the pan and heat cook for approximately 10 - 15 minutes (about 5 - 7 minutes per side). Season with salt and pepper.

3   In a large deep pan, boil some water and then add the cauliflower. Cook until soft and tender. Remove.

4   Add the broccoli and the celery to the pan and cook for an additional few more minutes, stir so it gets evenly cooked. Add more salt and pepper to the broccoli to taste.

5   Plate up the chicken and greens, adding the cauliflower.

Turkey & Peppers with Cauliflower Rice

Moderate-high in protein and *moderate* in fat
(Although carbohydrates are higher than the recommended consumption here, measurements are in total. For per serving, divide by 2)

CALORIES (KCAL): 560.5 | CARBS: 65.8G | PROTEIN: 51.9G | FAT: 23.5G
SERVES: 2 ADULTS

INGREDIENTS:

- ○ 4 x turkey steaks
- ○ ½ x red pepper
- ○ ½ x yellow pepper
- ○ ½ x green pepper
- ○ 8 x tomatoes
- ○ 1 ½ x cups mushrooms
- ○ 4 x ground garlic cloves
- ○ 1 x tbsp ground black pepper
- ○ ½ x tbsp cayenne
- ○ 2 x cups arugula

○ 1 x cups green beans

○ 1 x tbsp butter

○ 1 x cup low carb milk

METHOD:

1   Preheat the oven to around 190 degrees celsius. Line a baking tray with aluminium foil, place the turkey steaks on the tray and place the tray in the oven, cook for 20 - 30 minutes until the juices run clear when pierced, there are no pink bits, and the steaks are hot through.

2   Dice the peppers, tomatoes, mushrooms and grind the cloves. Place olive oil in a large pan and throw all of the vegetables in, as well as the arugula and garlic. Stir the vegetable mix until cooked.

3   Melt the butter in a deep pan, add the cauliflower rice and steadily stir while adding milk to the pan. Keep stirring until the cauliflower rice is rich and creamy, and then add the rest of milk and continue stirring. This should take around 15 - 18 minutes in total.

4   Remove the turkey steaks, placing two on each plate. Add the cauliflower rice and the vegetable mix proportionately, grab your utensils and enjoy!

Creamy Coconut Garlic Chicken

Moderate-high in protein and *high* in fat

**CALORIES (KCAL): 1,483 | CARBS: 37G | PROTEIN: 79G | FAT: 118G
SERVES: 2 ADULTS**

INGREDIENTS:

○ 2 x tbsp olive oil

○ 1 x spring onion

○ 4 x chicken breast fillets

○ 1 x cup coriander

○ ½ x tbsp salt

○ ⅓ x cup garlic powder

○ 1 x cup coconut cream

○ 1 x tsp paprika

○ 1 x tsp cumin

○ 1 x tsp ground ginger

○ 1 x cup parmesan cheese

O 4 x tomatoes

O ½ x tbsp ground black pepper

O ½ x tsp salt

METHOD:

1 In a large pan, cook the chicken fillets on a medium heat in olive oil for about 5 minutes per side. Cook until hot through, and so that no juices run when pierced. Remove the chicken from the pan and slice into strips or chunks (depending on preference) on an appropriate chopping board.

2 Using a deep, round, flat bowl, whisk together the coconut cream, paprika, parmesan cheese (microwaving if necessary - to soften the cheese), cumin, ground ginger and garlic powder, as well as the ground black pepper and salt.

3 Slice and dice the spring onion, tomatoes and place them in the pan (the one you used for the chicken should be fine) with additional olive oil. Cook until browning and then add the coconut cream goodness and continue stirring. Add the chicken, and then heat for an additional 8 - 10 minutes, adding the coriander.

4 Serve.

Keto Mac n Cheese

Moderate-high in protein and *very high* in fat
CALORIES (KCAL): 1,965 | CARBS: 19.3G | PROTEIN: 87.2G | FAT: 182.5G
SERVES: 2 ADULTS

INGREDIENTS:

○ 3 x tbsp olive oil

○ 4 x cups cheddar cheese (grated or shredded)

○ 1 x tbsp ground black pepper

○ 4 x tbsp cream cheese

○ 2 x cups mozzarella shredded

○ 2 x tbsp parmesan cheese

○ 1 x cup coconut cream

○ 2 x tbsp chopped parsley

○ 56g crackling

METHOD:

1 Preheat the oven to a medium heat. Chop up the cauliflower and place it in a bowl with the salt, pepper and oil and toss. Then, spread it on a baking tray and place in the oven, roasting it for around 40 minutes.

2 Pour the coconut cream into a pan and heat steadily on a medium heat. Bring it to a bowl, and then drop the temperature down again. Add the cheeses and stir until melted. Season the cream with salt and pepper and then add the roasted cauliflower.

3 Use a separate dish to prepare the crackling with the parmesan cheese and oil, mix together and then add to the cauliflower cheese dish. Stir for a while and then add the entire mixture to a baking dish, and bake until golden (15 - 20 minutes).

4 Garnish and then serve!

Coconut Curry Chicken with Cauliflower Rice

Moderate in protein and *high* in fat
(Measurements are in total, for per serving, divide by 3/4)
CALORIES (KCAL): 1,253 | CARBS: 50G | PROTEIN: 54G | FAT: 132G
SERVES: 3 - 4 ADULTS

INGREDIENTS:

○ 1 x spring onion

○ 1 x cup mushrooms

○ 2 x chicken breast fillets

○ 1 x red pepper diced

○ 3 x large tomatoes diced

○ 4 x tsp olive oil

○ 4 x ground garlic cloves

○ 1 x tsp paprika

○ 1 x cup coconut cream

- ◯ 3 x cups cauliflower rice

- ◯ 1 x cup low carb milk

- ◯ 1 x tsp cumin

- ◯ 1 x tsp ground ginger

- ◯ 1 x tbsp butter

METHOD:

1 Preheat the oven to a medium heat (around 190 degrees celsius). Lay a sheet of aluminium foil to a baking tray , place a drop of oil on the foil and spread across the tray. Add the chicken breasts to the tray and place the tray in the preheated oven. Cook for about 20 minutes.

2 Grind the garlic, slice and dice the tomatoes and peppers, quarter the onions, and slice the spring onion. Place another tsp of olive oil in a large pan and put the hob on a medium heat. Throw the sliced and diced spring onion into the pan and cook on a medium to high heat, until the spring onion slices begin to brown.

3 Remove the chicken, place it on an appropriate chopping board, and then add to the pan, adding also another tsp of olive oil. Stir the chicken with the spring onion, and then add the mushrooms, peppers and tomatoes. Stir the curry mix continuously, and then add the coconut cream. Keep stirring. Add the paprika, ginger and cumin.

4   Bring the curry mixture up to a boil, and then, finally, reduce the heat to a low heat and leave to simmer for 20 minutes or so, giving you a perfect opportunity to begin on the cauliflower rice!

5   Melt the butter in a deep pan, add the cauliflower rice and steadily stir while adding milk to the pan. Keep stirring until the cauliflower rice is rich and creamy, and then add the rest of milk and continue stirring. This should take around 15 - 18 minutes in total.

6   Plate up the rice as needed, and then add the curry to each plate as needed.

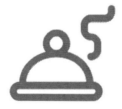

Side Dishes

It's late at night. You've had dinner but you're feeling peckish. Or, you're in between meals and are feeling like a snack. Or hell, you've had a great meal but you need a little pick me up or a dessert to really top it off. This is that important section of the book where we will give you some lowdons on snacks and desserts, debatably the most satisfying meal time for us who like a good midnight munch, or a satisfying dessert to see you home after a great meal. Based on what you have just read in the past few sentences, this section may look like the gluttonous enabling of overindulgent food habits, but that is far from the case. We believe that snacking is important. Not just because it can decrease hunger, and thus prevent eating too much at bigger meal times, but also because a good snack can be just enough to sustain without the weight gain. Snacks tide us over during busy periods, keeping us fuller for longer. They prevent us from feeling hungry at inconvenient times, and most importantly, they energise us when we need it. That snack you have mid afternoon before racing off to the gym will keep you grounded during this heavy session. Moreover, during working hours, a snack can be very important. We are all very busy and need sustenance from time to time, and a small bite can be just the ticket to tick us over into the next part of our day, without the need to stop and cook for an hour interrupting our busy schedules.

But also, desserts. There is something important to many of us about finding ways to replace the sweet stuff, and that is why we have included a selection of keto friendly desserts as well, so that you can make the transition fully without missing any of your favourite meal forms. Because let's face it, desserts are terrific, and that's not changing anytime soon.

And so, without further ado, here are a selection of ideas ranging from crunchy to healthy, and everything in between, that are sure to give you that well needed ballast, and send you speeding through the day with a mighty, energised passion, and give your mental health molecules something to munch on at the same time. Let's go!

Fried Asparagus Sticks

Low-moderate in protein and *very high* in fat
CALORIES (KCAL): 1087.8 | CARBS: 29.6G | PROTEIN: 20.54G | FAT: 117.1G
SERVES: 1-8 ADULTS

INGREDIENTS:

O 2 x tbsp olive oil

O 85 g unsweetened cashew milk

O 1 tbsp lemon juice

O 1 x tbsp ground paprika

O 1 ½ cup almond flour

O 1 x cups asparagus (not sliced)

O 1 ½ lemons zested

O 1 x cup macadamia nuts

METHOD:

1   Heat the olive oil in a pan on medium heat.

2   Mix the unsweetened cashew milk with the lemon juice. Stir thoroughly, adding the paprika, ground black pepper and salt (to taste) and then leave to sit for 8-10 minutes. Add the flour to a separate bowl.

3   Dip each asparagus in this buttermilk alternative mixture. Do them individually and then roll them in the macadamia nuts and flour. Coat rigorously.

4   Fry the coated asparagus in the pan for 8 - 10 minutes, until crispy and brown and serve.

Fried Avocado Chips with Salad

High in protein and *high* in fat
(Measurements are in total, for per serving, divide by 2)
**CALORIES (KCAL): 2,002 | CARBS: 63.7G | PROTEIN: 65G | FAT: 169G
SERVES: 2 ADULTS**

INGREDIENTS:

○ 4 x large eggs

○ 1 x tbs pouring cream

○ 2 x tsp table salt

○ 2 x tbsp ground black pepper

○ 2 x tsp paprika

○ 4 x avocados

○ 1 x cups grated cheddar cheese

○ 3 x cups almond meal

○ 1 ½ x cups ground macadamia nuts (for crunch)

○ 1 x lemon

○ 4 x tbsp tartare sauce

○ ¼ x tsp olive oil

○ 1 x cups arugula (rocket salad)

○ 1 x cups cherry tomatoes (sliced)

METHOD:

1 Preheat the oven to a medium heat. Line a baking tray with aluminium foil, covering in a light amount of olive oil.

2 Take the avocados and peel them, removing the stones and slicing them into wedges. If you are using 4 avocados, it will be 16 wedges in total.

3 Mix the eggs, pouring cream and 2 tbsp of water into a bowl. Whisk and rest. In a separate bowl, mix together the cheddar cheese, almond meal, macadamia nuts, paprika, black pepper and salt.

4 Coat the avocados in the egg mixture, and then douse them in a second coat of the almond meal, cheese and nut mixture. Allow the excess mixture to drip off of the slice and then place on the baking tray. Repeat this with every avocado slice and then place the baking tray in the oven for 20 - 25 minutes.

5   Assemble the rocket salad and tomatoes, pouring the tartare sauce into a separate ramekin for each plate, dispersing the salad mix evenly.

6   Once the avocado chips are done, remove them from the oven, and plate up the tasty, crunchy, and healthy snack, and enjoy!

Taco-cados!

(Measurements are in total, for per serving, divide by 12)
CALORIES (KCAL): 4,187 | CARBS: 129.59G | PROTEIN: 109.6G | FAT: 307G
SERVES: UP TO 12 ADULTS

INGREDIENTS:

- 6 x avocados

- 24 x cherry tomatoes

- 3 x cups ground beef

- 1 tsp garlic powder

- 1 tsp paprika

- 2 x cans chopped tomatoes

- 1 x spring onion

- ½ x red pepper

- 1 x cup lime juice

- 1 tsp salt

- ½ tbsp ground black pepper

○ 1 tsp cumin

○ 2 x cups cheddar cheese

○ 1 x tbsp olive oil

METHOD:

1 Heat olive oil in a large pan. Slice and dice the spring onion, pepper and half the cherry tomatoes. Place the spring onion in the large pan and cook until browning, adding all of the vegetables at the browned stage. Add the ground beef, garlic powder, salt, ground black pepper and cumin, and cook until hot and then add both cans of chopped tomatoes. Continue to stir, adding the lime juice last.

2 Half the avocados, remove the stones, and remove some of the avocado from the middle and place in a separate bowl (so you can fit more filling in). You can use the discarded avocado to make some taste bud tantalising guacamole for your side dish!

3 Using a slotted spoon, scoop the beef mix from the pan and fill the avocados, adding plenty of parmesan cheese to the top.

4 Plate up the avocados and serve to up to 12 guests (or, just have them all to yourself. I would.) Use a spoon, and do not eat the skin.

Keto Double Chocolate Chip Brownies

(Measurements are in total, for per serving, divide by 5)

CALORIES (KCAL): 1,522 | CARBS: 201G | PROTEIN: 34.5G | FAT: 104G
SERVES: 5 ADULTS

INGREDIENTS:

○ 1 x cups almond flour

○ 2 x cups erythritol

○ 3 x cups cocoa powder

○ 1 x tsp bicarbonate of soda

○ 2 x tbsp butter

○ 2 x tbsp low carb milk e.g almond milk

○ 2 x cups chocolate chips (optional but simply delicious)

○ 2 x large eggs

METHOD:

1 Using a deep, round bowl, mix together the almond flour, erythritol, cocoa powder and bicarbonate of soda (the dry ingredients). Mix until fused together well.

2 In a separate bowl, whisk the butter with the 2 large eggs and milk until the three ingredients are fused well.

3 Put the second mixture into the dry ingredients mixture and whisk all ingredients together, adding the chocolate chips if using these (alchemy!).

4 PLay out your brownie mix in an appropriate baking tray and preheat the oven to about 190 degrees celsius, insert the brownie mix and bake for 20 - 25 minutes until risen and looking delicious and chocolatey.

5 Cut and serve as required. Enjoy!

Cinnamon Whirls

(Measurements are in total. For per serving divide by 12)
CALORIES (KCAL): 2,045 | CARBS: 10.4G | PROTEIN: 73.7G | FAT: 162G
SERVES: UP TO 12 ADULTS

INGREDIENTS:

○ 4 x tbsp butter

○ 1 x tbsp cinnamon

○ 2 x tbsp tap water

○ 1 x tsp bicarbonate of soda

○ 1 x cup almond flour

○ ½ x cup erythritol (or your preferred sugar mix substitute)

○ 1 x large egg

○ 2 x tbsp cream cheese

○ 2 x cups grated cheese (e.g mozzarella)

METHOD:

1 Place the grated cheese with the cream cheese in a deep, round plastic bowl. Melt them together in the microwave for approximately 30 - 60 seconds so that they meld together. Add the egg, flour, erythritol sugar mix substitute and bicarbonate of soda and whisk all of these ingredients together. Continue until you have a thick, sturdy dough.

2 Mix the butter, cinnamon, and erythritol in a separate bowl. Roll out the dough into a large square (use a good size rolling pin) and spread the mixture over it. Then, laying the dough out flat, roll it into a log shape. It is advisable at this point to refrigerate the dough roll for approximately 30 minutes in order to harden it slightly, and thus, it will be sturdier when cut. Slice the log into 12 separate pieces using a dough divider or a large knife.

3 Preheat the oven to about 190 degrees celsius. Place each unbaked cinnamon whirl on the baking tray. Bake for 12 - 15 minutes until the colour of freshly mined gold.

4 Mix a cup of erythritol with water in a jug or glass, mix with a spoon until icing forms. Refrigerate for 10 minutes or so. Remove the freshly baked cinnamon whirls from the oven, and spread the icing over each one.

5   Serve and snack at your leisure.

Shrewsbury Biscuits

CALORIES (KCAL): 3,098 | CARBS: 22G | PROTEIN: 20G | FAT: 206.2G
SERVES: 1 - 12 ADULTS

INGREDIENTS:

○ 2 x large eggs

○ 1 ½ cups butter

○ 2 ½ x cups almond flour

○ 1 ½ x cups erythritol

○ 2 x tbsp cinnamon

METHOD:

1. Using a round, flat, deep bowl (optimally plastic), pour in the almond flour, erythritol, butter and cinnamon, adding the eggs and whisking, optimally with an electric whisk, so as to speed the process up. If you are using a fork it can still be done, it just takes longer.

2. Preheat the oven. Lay out the biscuit dough, rolling it flat on a wooden surface (e.g a chopping board) and use a biscuit slicer to cut the dough into appropriate, consistent sizes. Take two or more baking trays and line them with aluminium foil. Carefully place your sliced cake shapes and place them on the trays.

3. Bake in the oven for 10 - 15 minutes until risen and golden brown.

4. Serve and consume while warm, soft and delicious!

Disclaimer

This book contains opinions and ideas of the author and is meant to teach the reader informative and helpful knowledge while due care should be taken by the user in the application of the information provided. The instructions and strategies are possibly not right for every reader and there is no guarantee that they work for everyone. Using this book and implementing the information/ recipes therein contained is explicitly your own responsibility and risk. This work with all its contents, does not guarantee correctness, completion, quality or correctness of the provided information. Misinformation or misprints cannot be completely eliminated.

Printed in Great Britain
by Amazon

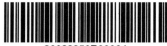